CW01209392

High Blood Pressure: Your Quick Guide to Understanding and Treatment

ISBN-13: 978-1489529480
ISBN-10: 1489529489

Copyright Notice

All Rights Reserved © 2013 Edward Freingard

This book is a work of the author's experience and opinion. This book is licensed for your personal enjoyment only. This book may not be re-sold or given away to other people. If you would like to share this book with another person please purchase an additional copy for each person you share it with. You may not distribute or sell this book or modify it in any way. The editorial arrangement, analysis, and professional commentary are subject to this copyright notice. No portion of this book may be copied, retransmitted, reposted, downloaded, decompiled, reverse engineered, duplicated, or otherwise used without the express written approval of the author, except by reviewers who may quote brief excerpts in connection with a review. The scanning, uploading and distribution of this book via the internet or via any other means without permission of the publisher is illegal and punishable by law. The publisher does not have any control over and does not assume any responsibility for author or third-party websites or their content. United States laws and regulations are public domain and not subject to copyright. Any unauthorized copying, reproduction, translation, or distribution of any part of this material without permission by the author is prohibited and against the law. Disclaimer and Terms of Use: No information contained in this book should be considered as financial, tax, or legal advice. Your reliance upon information and content obtained by you at or through this publication is solely at your own risk. The authors or publishers assume no liability or responsibility for damage or injury to you, other persons, or property arising from any use of any product, information, idea, or instruction contained in the content or services provided to you through this book. Reliance upon information contained in this material is solely at the reader's own risk. The authors have no financial interest in and receive no compensation from manufacturers of products or websites mentioned in this book. Whilst attempts have been made to verify information provided in this publication, neither the author nor the publisher assumes any responsibilities for errors, omissions or contradictory information contained in this book. The author and publisher make no representation or warranties with respect to the accuracy, applicability, fitness, or completeness of the contents of this book. The information contained in this book is strictly for educational purposes. The author and publisher do not warrant the performance, effectiveness or applicability of any information or sites listed or linked to in this book.

HIGH BLOOD PRESSURE: YOUR QUICK GUIDE TO UNDERSTANDING AND TREATMENT

Edward Freingard

To those who have suffered with the time bomb that is high blood pressure. I hope the information here helps bring some comfort to your life.

Contents

1. An Overview of High Blood Pressure
2. Symptoms of High Blood Pressure
3. Causes of High Blood Pressure
4. Risk Factors Associated with High Blood Pressure
5. Possible Complications of High Blood Pressure
6. Preventing High Blood Pressure
7. High Blood Pressure: Preparing for an Appointment
8. Blood Pressure Tests and Diagnosis
9. Hypertension Treatment: Go Natural
10. Lifestyle Changes toHelp Reduce High Blood Pressure
11. Natural Remedies for High Blood Pressure
12. Herbal Remedies and a Holistic Approach
13. What Part Does Potassium Play?
14. The Food Factor
15. Living with High Blood Pressure

An Overview of High Blood Pressure

As you may already be aware of, high blood pressure is often a precursor to coronary heart disease, stroke, heart attacks, and even kidney failure.

If you ever hope to spare yourself from the condition, then the best way to begin is by understanding exactly what high blood pressure is.

To begin with, the term 'blood pressure' refers to the force of your blood as it pushes against your arterial walls while your heart continues to pump blood.

This pressure needs to stay at a healthy level; otherwise, significant damage can occur in a lot of ways. Perhaps the saddest thing about high blood pressure is that it is very prevalent.

In the United States alone, one out of every three adults has the condition.

Another concern is the fact that the condition seldom shows any symptoms until your blood pressure has become extremely high.

The fact that it has practically no symptoms means your heart, kidneys, blood vessels, and other organs could already have been damaged without your knowledge.

This is why it's important for you to always be aware of your blood pressure numbers. If you have normal blood pressure, then you need to do whatever you can to maintain that.

If you find that your blood pressure is already too high, then you need work on lowering it as soon as possible to prevent damage to any of your body's organs.

Your blood pressure is typically measured according to the systolic and diastolic pressures. Systolic pressure is the pressure of your blood when your heart beats as it pumps blood.

Diastolic pressure is the pressure of your blood while your heart is at rest in-between beats. When you hear that your blood pressure is 120 over 80 (written as 120/80 mmHg), it means your systolic pressure is 120mmHg and your diastolic pressure is 80mmHg.

Take note that normal systolic pressure for adults is below 120 and normal diastolic pressure is below 80. Blood pressure of 120/80 is therefore borderline and anything above that is abnormally high.

Remember, though, that it's normal for a person's blood pressure to vary at different times of day.

Your blood pressure will normally lower as you sleep and rise upon waking up. It's also normal for your blood pressure to rise when you're nervous, active, or excited.

But, if your blood pressure is high almost all the time, then it's definitely time to consult your doctor and get properly diagnosed.

In case your systolic pressure is high, but your diastolic pressure is still within normal range, take note that you're still considered as having high blood pressure and will therefore need to take the necessary steps to get your blood pressure under control.

The risk for high blood pressure rises with age. The good thing is that a healthy lifestyle can help prevent high blood pressure or at least delay the onset.

And if you already have high blood pressure, leading a healthy lifestyle can help you keep it under control, along with treatment and ongoing medical care.

Symptoms of
High Blood Pressure

People often think that they'll know when they have high blood pressure because they're likely to experience such symptoms as sweating, nervousness, facial flushes, and difficulty in sleeping.

The truth, however, is that high blood pressure only shows symptoms when you already have hypertensive crisis, which means your blood pressure is already dangerously high.

Therefore, don't be too complacent simply because you think there are symptoms that'll alert you to the condition.

Be sure to check your blood pressure regularly and take the necessary steps to prevent high blood pressure instead.

Headaches

It was previously believed that headaches were common in those who suffer from high blood pressure.

The truth is that headaches are common only in people who have hypertensive crisis.

In fact, a study has shown that headaches are less common in people with high blood pressure as compared to the general population.

The study also shows that when your systolic pressure is higher than normal, you're 40% less likely to experience headaches.

Additionally, people with a higher pulse pressure than normal are 50% less likely to experience headaches.

Headaches or the lack of it isn't a reliable indicator of high blood pressure and it's still advisable to keep track of your blood pressure numbers.

Nosebleeds

Again, only those who suffer from hypertensive crisis are likely to have nosebleeds as an indicator.

Although it has indeed been noted that people with high blood pressure have more nosebleeds than those with normal pressure, this is not really a reliable indicator, since there could be a variety of other explanations for the nosebleed.

It's best to consult your doctor if you experience frequent nosebleeds or if your nosebleed is heavy and difficult to stop.

Dry air, colds, sinusitis, allergies, and vigorous blowing of your nose are common causes of nosebleeds.

Other Symptoms

Other conditions that are commonly believed to be symptoms of high blood pressure, but aren't really reliable indicators include blood spots in your eyes, facial flushes, and dizziness.

It's true that blood spots are common in people with high blood pressure, but it's also common in those who suffer from diabetes.

More importantly, neither condition directly causes blood spots. It's best to get your eyes checked by an ophthalmologist.

Where facial flushing is concerned, there are indeed times when it occurs while your blood pressure is high, but that's only because some of the things that cause facial flushing can also cause a rise in blood pressure.

These include emotional stress, alcohol consumption, exercise, and exposure to extreme heat or cold.

As for dizziness, it isn't really a symptom of high blood pressure, but a common side effect of some medications for the condition. This doesn't mean you should ignore dizziness, of course.

Remember that sudden dizziness coupled with a loss of coordination or balance is usually a warning sign for stroke.

Where high blood pressure is concerned, it's important that you avoid evaluating your symptoms on your own.

Self-diagnosis is never advised for this condition. Rather, you should keep track of your blood pressure and then consult your doctor as soon as possible if you notice that your blood pressure is rising more often than normal.

Causes of High Blood Pressure

Even in this day and age when the condition has become so prevalent, the things that cause high blood pressure directly still aren't known.

However, a number of factors and conditions have been identified and determined to play a major role in the development of the condition.

These include smoking, obesity, inactivity, stress, old age, genetics, too much alcohol, too much salt consumption, thyroid and adrenal disorders, and kidney disease.

Take note that the direct cause of about 95% of high blood pressure cases cannot be determined. This phenomenon is referred to as essential hypertension.

As mentioned earlier, studies have linked it to a number of risk factors, though its exact causes remain mysterious.

High blood pressure generally runs in families and men are more commonly affected than women.

Your age and race are also likely to play a major role. In the case of the United States, for example, whites are only half as likely as blacks to suffer from the condition.

Your lifestyle and diet are also very influential in terms of your likelihood to suffer from essential hypertension.

You should take special note of the link between the condition and your salt intake.

For instance, people living in Northern Japan consume more salt than any other group of people in the world.

They also have the world's highest recorded incidence of essential hypertension.

In contrast to this observation, those who consume practically no salt show almost no trace of essential hypertension.

Bear in mind that every single sufferer of high blood pressure is known to be salt sensitive.

This means that when they take in more salt than the minimum amount needed by the human body, their blood pressure will immediately increase.

Other than salt and the risk factors mentioned above, you risk of suffering from essential hypertension also increases as a result of stress, lack of potassium intake, inactivity, lack of calcium, too much alcohol, lack of magnesium, obesity, and diabetes.

In the rare event that the direct cause of high blood pressure is identified, the condition is known as secondary hypertension.

Kidney disease is the most common known cause of high blood pressure.

Other than that, though, you may also suffer from high blood pressure resulting from tumors and other abnormalities that may cause your adrenal glands to secrete too much of the hormones that normally raise a person's blood pressure.

Pregnancy, medications that result in blood vessel constriction, and birth control pills that contain estrogen are also known to increase blood pressure.

Now that you know more about what could possibly raise your blood pressure, you'd do well to avoid these factors and conditions as much as you can.

Of course, there's nothing you can do about your genetic make-up, but being aware that your genetics could very well be a risk factor for high blood pressure gives you the opportunity to take the necessary precautions.

Take stock of your current lifestyle and determine if you're inadvertently putting yourself at risk for hypertension.

If so, then it's definitely a good idea to start making positive changes right now.

Risk Factors Associated with High Blood Pressure

There are several risk factors for high blood pressure and you'd do well to avoid them as much as you can.

These risk factors include certain conditions, habits, and traits.

And while you may not be able to do anything about some of them, you can still do much to prevent or at least delay the onset of high blood pressure.

Naturally, it pays to know what the risk factors are.

Age

Blood pressure normally rises as you age. This may be why more than half of the world's senior citizens have high blood pressure.

In most cases where the condition is brought about by age, it is the systolic pressure that ranks abnormally high.

In fact, about two-thirds of those who suffer from high blood pressure due to age have what is known as isolated systolic hypertension.

Take note, though, that high blood pressure isn't considered a normal part of the aging process.

There are plenty of ways for you to stay healthy as you age and you need to take advantage of these ways.

Ethnicity and Race

While practically anyone can develop high blood pressure, there are those who are more at risk because of their race and ethnicity.

African Americans, for example, are more likely to develop the condition than Hispanics or Caucasians.

Additionally, African Americans also have a tendency to develop high blood pressure earlier in life and their cases are usually more severe.

The good news is that they're also more aware of their risk for high blood pressure and are more willing to seek treatment.

Among Hispanic groups, Puerto Ricans are known to be more likely to develop the condition than others.

Obesity

If you're obese or even just overweight, your risk for developing high blood pressure is also increased.

Be sure to take note of what your ideal weight is and then strive to achieve and maintain that weight.

Gender

Adult men are more likely to suffer from high blood pressure than women, but adult women are more likely to seek treatment for the condition than men.

Men only become more likely to seek treatment when they reach the age of 60.

But when adults reach this age, men are more likely to gain control of their blood pressure than women.

Lifestyle

Take note that certain habits are known risk factors for high blood pressure.

Therefore, if you already have some of the other risk factors mentioned above, you should be sure to avoid consuming too much salt, drinking too much alcohol, and smoking.

You should also make sure you take in an adequate amount of potassium and engage in regular exercise.

Other risk factors for the condition include a family history of high blood pressure. If you're subjected to stressful situations in a prolonged manner, then you're also more likely to suffer from the condition.

Knowing all these, you should realize the importance of getting your blood pressure checked regularly if you have any of the above-mentioned risk factors.

Remember that keeping your blood pressure at normal levels saves you from developing serious health problems that may put your life at risk.

Possible Complications of High Blood Pressure

High blood pressure causes excessive pressure on the walls of your arteries and this pressure can cause some serious damage to your blood vessels and major organs.

The higher your blood pressure is and the longer you allow it to remain that way, the greater the damage it can cause.

Among the possible complications that can result from high blood pressure that remains unchecked are the following:

1. **Heart Attack or Stroke**

    When you leave high blood pressure untreated and uncontrolled, it can cause your arteries to thicken and harden, thus leading to atherosclerosis. This condition, in turn, can cause a heart attack or stroke, or some other type of complication.

2. **Aneurysm**

    When your blood pressure is increased, your blood vessels can weaken and bulge, thus leading to the formation of an aneurysm.

In the event that this aneurysm ruptures, your life can hang in the balance.

3. **Weakened Blood Vessels in the Kidneys**

   High blood pressure can weaken the blood vessels in your kidneys, thus preventing the organ from functioning as it should.

4. **Heart Failure**

   Your heart naturally works harder when it tries to pump blood against higher pressure. It thickens as a result and starts having a hard time pumping enough blood for your body's daily needs. This situation can soon lead to heart failure.

5. **Metabolic Syndrome**

   This refers to a cluster of disorders associated with your metabolism, including an increase in the circumference of your waist, low levels of good cholesterol, high levels of triglycerides, and high levels of insulin.

Having high blood pressure increases your likelihood of experiencing the various components of metabolic syndrome. Take note that the more of these components you experience, the higher your risk for diabetes, stroke, and heart disease will be.

6. **Memory and Comprehension Problems**

   If you leave high blood pressure untreated and uncontrolled, your ability to think, understand, learn, and remember may also be negatively affected. Studies have shown that people with high blood pressure are more likely to experience problems with memory and understanding.

7. **Narrowed, Thickened, or Torn Blood Vessels in Your Eyes**

   If you allow your hypertension to become so severe as to cause blood vessels in your eyes to thicken, become narrowed, or get torn, then you could be in danger of losing your vision.

Now that you're aware of what possible complications may arise from high blood pressure, you should realize how important it is to keep your blood pressure at a healthy level.

Be sure to check if you have any of the risk factors for the condition and then do your best to take the necessary precautions.

Things like age and genetics may be something you can't do anything about, but risk factors like lifestyle are definitely under your control.

It is also a good idea to have your blood pressure checked on a regular basis to make sure you're successfully keeping it at normal levels.

In case your blood pressure remains high for several days, get yourself tested and diagnosed by your doctor immediately.

Preventing High Blood Pressure

High blood pressure is considered a major risk factor for kidney disease, heart failure, stroke, and heart disease. The fact that it generally shows no symptoms makes it all the more dangerous.

The good thing is that it's easy enough to find out if you have the condition simply by checking your blood pressure on a regular basis. If your blood pressure is high, then you can take the necessary steps to lower it.

If it is normal, then you can take the necessary steps to keep it that way. Among the ways you can avoid high blood pressure are the following:

1. **Maintain a Healthy Weight**

    If you are overweight, then you are at least twice more likely to develop hypertension than if you are at your ideal weight.

    Take note that even the tiniest amount of weight that you lose can make a huge difference in your efforts to hold hypertension at bay.

2. **Exercise Regularly**

   Active individuals generally have a significantly lower risk of developing high blood pressure than those who are inactive.

   Of course, this doesn't mean you have to be a serious athlete in order to avoid hypertension. It only means you need to engage in even the lightest of exercises, like walking, on a daily basis.

3. **Keep Salt Intake at a Minimum**

   Cutting back on your salt intake has been shown to prevent high blood pressure. Conversely, a high salt intake has been linked to increased risk for high blood pressure.

4. **Drink Moderately**

   You hear this in liquor commercials all the time. If you want to avoid hypertension, then it's definitely a good idea to take heed of the warning. Two drinks a day should suffice for men, while one drink each day is advised for women.

5. **Keep Stress at Bay**

   Stress is one of the most common culprits in cases of high blood pressure.

   The good thing is that there are plenty of ways for you to avoid stress. Try some relaxation techniques and then apply those that work best on you.

You may also be able to prevent the development of high blood pressure if you increase your intake of the following nutrients:

1. **Potassium**

   Fish, dairy products, and most fresh fruits and vegetables are excellent sources of potassium.

   It's a good thing that it's easy to get enough potassium from food sources because taking supplements without your doctor's supervision can be a bit dangerous.

2. **Calcium**

   People who lack calcium intake have been shown to have high rates of hypertension, although it hasn't been proven that supplementing with calcium tablets can effectively prevent the condition.

   Of course, there's no harm in making sure you get enough calcium each day. Low-fat milk, cheese, and yogurt are excellent sources of calcium.

3. **Magnesium**

   Just like potassium, you can get enough magnesium from your diet and doctors don't really advise taking extra magnesium supplements.

   What you need to do instead is increase your intake of whole grains, nuts, seeds, green leafy vegetables, dry beans, and peas.

4. **Fish Oils**

   Omega-3 fatty acids, which is normally found in fatty fish such as salmon and mackerel is known to help reduce blood pressure.

   Take note, though, that high doses of fish oil can have unpleasant side effects, so avoid taking supplements.

5. **Garlic**

   Not only does garlic reduce your blood pressure, but it also improves your cholesterol levels and reduces your risk for some cancers.

Be sure to consult your doctor before taking any dietary supplement or medication for hypertension. It's best to consume the necessary nutrients direct from food sources.

High Blood Pressure: Preparing for an Appointment

If you check your blood pressure on a daily basis and you notice that it has been high for a few days, be sure to set an appointment with your doctor immediately so you can be properly diagnosed.

The good thing about this kind of appointment is that you don't need to make any special preparations.

It may be a good idea to wear a short-sleeved shirt to make it easier for the doctor to fit the blood pressure cuff around your arm.

Perhaps the only preparation you need to make is to use the toilet before your blood pressure is measured.

Remember that a number of medications like antidepressants, cold medicine, and birth control pills tend to raise your blood pressure.

This makes it important for you to list down any medication you may currently be taking and then bring the list when you see your doctor.

Don't just stop taking any medication because you think it will affect your blood pressure. Be sure to seek advice from your doctor first.

Doctor's appointments are often brief, so you'll have to be prepared for it to make sure you cover everything that needs to be covered.

One of the things you can do in preparation for a doctor's appointment is to write down all symptoms you may be experiencing.

Although high blood pressure generally has no symptoms, it's a good idea to list down anything you may be feeling that's out of the ordinary.

This will make it easier for your doctor to gauge the level of aggressiveness with which your condition should be treated.

It also pays to write down important personal information such as major stresses in your life or any recent change you've been through.

Any family history of hypertension, heart disease, high cholesterol, stroke, or diabetes should also be noted.

Additionally, you'd do well to list down any medication, vitamins, or dietary supplements you may be taking.

You may also want to bring a family member or friend along, not just for moral support, but also to help you take in all the information provided by your doctor.

Furthermore, you have to be prepared to openly discuss your dietary and exercise habits with your doctor.

Take note that you may have to make some adjustments in this regard, depending on the doctor's diagnosis of your condition. It's also a good idea to write down any questions you may have for your doctor to make sure everything about your condition is clear to you.

Just as you've prepared some questions to ask your doctor, you can also expect your doctor to ask you a number of questions.

As mentioned above, he is likely to ask about your family history of high blood pressure, heart disease, and high cholesterol. He is also likely to ask if you smoke or drink alcohol regularly.

Additionally, your doctor will likely ask when you last had your blood pressure checked and what result you got at that time.

While waiting for your appointment, you may want to start making some healthy lifestyle changes.

Blood Pressure Tests and Diagnosis

A person's blood pressure is typically measured with the use of a sphygmomanometer. The measurement is given in mmHg or millimetres of mercury.

The first number given is the systolic pressure, which is the arterial pressure as your heart beats.

The second number given is the diastolic pressure, which is the arterial pressure after each heartbeat.

There are generally four categories into which the measurement of blood pressure falls and these are the following:

1. **Normal**

    If your blood pressure has a measurement of below 120/80 mmHg, then it is still within the normal range. There are doctors, however, who recommend that you aim for a blood pressure of 115/75 mmHg instead.

That's because the risk for cardiovascular disease starts to rise the moment your blood pressure goes beyond this measurement.

2. **Pre-hypertension**

    When your systolic pressure reaches 120-139 mmHg or your diastolic pressure measures 80-89 mmHg, you are said to be in a pre-hypertension stage. Even if you still don't have hypertension at this stage, it's still important to lower your blood pressure because pre-hypertension tends to grow worse when ignored.

3. **Stage 1 Hypertension**

    You have Stage 1 hypertension when your systolic pressure has reached 140-159 mmHg or your diastolic pressure measures 90-99 mmHg. Needless to say, you'll have to get your condition treated at this point.

4. **Stage 2 Hypertension**

    When your systolic pressure has reached 160 mmHg or higher or your diastolic pressure measures 100 mmHg or higher, then you already have severe hypertension and will definitely need treatment and close supervision from your doctor.

Take note that your systolic and diastolic pressures are both important, so you need to keep track of them both. When you're over the age of 50, though, systolic pressure becomes a lot more significant.

That's because a condition known as isolated systolic hypertension becomes most common at this age.

This condition arises when you have normal diastolic pressure, but your systolic pressure is abnormally high.

It is likely that your doctor will take about three readings of your blood pressure during an appointment and he is also likely to set up at least two appointments with you so as to arrive at a proper diagnosis.

The reason for this is that a person's blood pressure normally varies at different times during the day. For some individuals, it's even normal for the blood pressure to rise during visits to their doctor.

This is something known as white-coat hypertension. Your doctor may even ask you to measure your blood pressure at work and at home so he'll have more specific information.

If your doctor finds that you have high blood pressure of any type, then he may recommended a number of routine tests like urinalysis, electrocardiogram, and some blood tests.

Additionally, he may recommend a cholesterol test and any other test he deems important to check for any sign of heart disease.

It is indeed very important for you to regularly monitor your blood pressure at home so you'll know when it's time to see your doctor for proper diagnosis and treatment.

You can ask your doctor for advice on how to properly measure your blood pressure if you're not sure.

Hypertension Treatment: Go Natural

High blood pressure or hypertension is among the most common medical conditions in the world. You may not realize it, but a diagnosis of high blood pressure is a serious thing.

In fact, it is the cause of thousands of deaths each year that are associated with heart disease, heart attack, kidney complications, and stroke.

The problem becomes even more serious when you consider the fact that the numbers rise each year as more and more people suffer from the condition.

And because the number keeps rising, people are looking for more ways of dealing with high blood pressure.

Although there are various treatment methods for high blood pressure, it may be a good idea to go natural and turn to home remedies. One of the biggest advantages of going natural is that you won't have to deal with the rising prices of prescription drugs.

Furthermore, the availability of these drugs isn't always assured whereas home remedies are in abundance.

Pharmaceutical drugs also continue to be associated with side effects when taken in the long-term, so you're definitely better off treating high blood pressure naturally.

Nature has provided us with the gift of herbs that can boost the function of your body's various systems. More importantly, a number of these herbs serve to naturally strengthen your heart.

At present, several scientific studies have proven some plants and herbs effective in normalizing a person's blood pressure.

Herbal medicines have even been formulated from these scientifically-proven plant sources.

The biggest advantage of herbal medicines is that they're associated with fewer side effects, thus making them a lot safer than prescription drugs.

It's a fact that once you're diagnosed with high blood pressure, you'll have to deal with it for life. This means you'll have to take medications on a regular basis and make lifetime adjustments to your habits and lifestyle.

The problem with some prescription drugs is that using them for the long-term can increase your risk of developing side effects or complications.

Natural remedies, on the other hand, have fewer side effects and aren't known to cause or aggravate complications, which is why it's generally a better option. Natural remedies for high blood pressure are also a lot less expensive than prescription drugs, which makes them more financially accessible.

Availability is also another huge advantage of natural remedies. You don't need prescription for them and you can even grow some herbs like pepper and garlic at home. Herbal medication therefore makes health a lot more accessible to the general public.

Cayenne pepper and garlic are among the most popular home remedies for high blood pressure.

Garlic, for one, has been used for years as an anti-cholesterol herb and is also deemed the top herb for hypertension. It has properties that help reduce bad cholesterol and lipids in your blood, thus protecting your heart.

Cayenne pepper, for its part, is the top herb for promoting proper blood circulation. These and other herbs used to treat high blood pressure work best when used hand-in-hand with water.

That's because a properly hydrated body naturally has good blood quality and circulation.

Hydration is also essential for flushing out inorganic salts and harmful toxins from your body.

Be sure to drink a minimum of eight glasses of water each day. The moment you become diagnosed with high blood pressure, bear in mind that it's better to go natural than to choose prescription drugs.

Lifestyle Changes to Help Reduce High Blood Pressure

Common treatment methods for high blood pressure include medication and lifestyle changes. The goal is for you to achieve and maintain a blood pressure lower than 140/90 mmHg.

Among the lifestyle changes you need to make in hopes of maintaining a healthy blood pressure is to start eating a healthy diet and exercising regularly.

You should strive to achieve and maintain your ideal body weight. If you're a smoker, then you'd do well to quit the habit. You should also learn how to deal with stress in a healthy manner.

Take note that doing all of the measures mentioned above is so much better than taking one measure alone.

Understandably, major lifestyle changes are difficult to make, but if you make the adjustments gradually, then the necessary changes can be made without too much difficulty.

If you're not that old yet, then it may be possible to keep your blood pressure under control with lifestyle changes alone. This means you may not really need medication. Even if you do need to take medication, take note that it's still important to make healthy lifestyle changes.

To begin with, you'll have to start eating a healthy diet. Your doctor will most probably recommend eating more fruits and vegetables as well as whole grains and other foods with low sodium content.

A diet plan known as DASH is often recommended, as it is low in cholesterol and fat, and focuses on food choices that are generally good for the heart.

Fish, poultry, nuts, low-fat milk, and dairy products are the usual components of this diet plan.

It also involves eating less red meat, sweets, and beverages rich in sugar. In general, it is rich in nutrients, fibre, and protein.

Another important lifestyle change you need to make so as to keep your blood pressure under control is to start exercising regularly.

Senior adults often think they're too old for exercise. That's not necessarily true. You'd do well to seek advice from your doctor as regards the types of exercise you can safely do and how much exercise you need.

Even simple activities like walking, riding a bicycle, working in your garden, cleaning your house, bowling, and dancing can do much to improve your blood pressure.

If your doctor gives you the go signal, then you may also want to consider swimming, jogging, and recreational sports.

Smoking has been known to damage blood vessels and increase the risk for high blood pressure. It can even aggravate the health problems commonly associated with high blood pressure. This is therefore another major adjustment smokers have to make.

If you really want to keep your blood pressure under control, then you'll have to quit. Your doctor can offer advice regarding products and programs that can help you quit the dangerous habit of smoking.

Another thing that can help you keep your blood pressure within a healthy range is learning to manage stress.

You may want to learn some relaxation techniques or unwind through physical activity.

Music may also help you relax and clear your mind. Whatever you choose to do, don't forget to measure your blood pressure regularly.

Natural Remedies for High Blood Pressure

Keeping your blood pressure under control is one of the best things you can ever do for your own health. There have been a lot of cases where people didn't know that had problems with their blood pressure simply because the condition generally has no physical symptoms. Bear in mind that when you have high blood pressure, your risk for suffering from a heart attack is increased. High blood pressure also causes damage not only to your heart, but to your kidneys and cells as well. This makes it all the more important for you to check your blood pressure on a regular basis.

When you're diagnosed with high blood pressure, you'll typically be given some prescription. But, remember that it's not really advisable to depend on drugs for controlling your blood pressure. It is more advantageous for you to make some positive changes in your dietary habits and lifestyle in general. A rise in your blood pressure can be caused by your daily problems and stresses. Take note that your systolic pressure (upper number) should not go beyond 140 and your diastolic pressure (lower number) should not go over 90. Once it does, you'll need to set up a doctor's appointment immediately for proper diagnosis and treatment.

The good news is that there are a number of natural ways for you to control your blood pressure.

One of these ways is to take coQ10 supplements, as this substance has been shown to improve blood pressure numbers. Another effective natural remedy for high blood pressure is garlic.

You can take garlic as is with your food or in supplement form. Take note, though, that you need to consult your doctor before supplementing with garlic, as this may interact with other medications and supplements.

Hawthorn is also one of the herbs commonly used by traditional medicine practitioners to treat high blood pressure. The good thing about hawthorn is that there are no known interactions.

Fish oil supplements may also be good for those who suffer from high blood pressure. Studies have shown that these supplements contain EPA and DHA.

DHA has previously been shown to help lower blood pressure. Folic acid or folate is a type of Vitamin B that is known to help form red blood cells in your body. This is important for lowering your blood pressure because it reduces the levels of homocystenine in your body.

All of the natural remedies for high blood pressure mentioned above are in the form of food or dietary supplements. Of course, there are also some lifestyle changes you can use to effectively keep your blood pressure in check.

First of all, you should strive to achieve and maintain your ideal weight by exercising regularly and following a healthy diet plan.

Among the things you need to adjust in your diet is your salt intake. Take note that too much salt intake increases your blood pressure, so be sure to keep your salt consumption at a minimum.

You should also stop smoking and reduce your alcohol consumption.

Bear in mind that your habits where eating, sleeping, and lifestyle are concerned have a direct effect on whatever disease or disorder you may be suffering from.

Working on these aspects, therefore, is the best way for you to improve your health.

Herbal Remedies and a Holistic Approach

A natural and holistic approach can definitely do much to lower your blood pressure and improve your cardiovascular health. This natural approach necessarily involves making positive lifestyle changes and using scientifically-proven herbal remedies.

If you've led an inactive lifestyle before, then starting an exercise regimen that involves as little as 30 minutes of activity each day can already have an immediate positive effect on your blood pressure.

Furthermore, losing just ten pounds of excess weight will make a huge difference in your health.

Small changes in your eating habits such as putting in a little more garlic and other herbs while reducing the salt are also known to have significantly beneficial effects.

You may also appreciate knowing that the polyphenols found in teas can help prevent the build-up of plaque in your arteries and veins. By drinking two to three cups of hibiscus tea or green tea each day, you can effectively lower your blood pressure.

Even herbal diuretics can have a positive effect, since they are known to eliminate edema. The herb Angelica is known to contain compounds that can serve as calcium channel blockers.

You're probably aware of the fact that blockers are commonly prescribed to promote heart health and treat high blood pressure. Some studies have also shown that Nigel la has a positive effect on blood pressure.

Aromatherapy has also been recognized as an effective treatment option for high blood pressure.

It is lauded because of its relaxing effect and the fact that it helps free you from the tension and stress that can contribute to your high blood pressure.

Recommended hypotensive oils include ylang-ylang, lavender, and marjoram. You can use these stabilizing oils and herbs when you draw a bath, in the form of a mist spray, or when getting a therapeutic massage.

You may have heard that plants containing berberine are very effective for treating intestinal disorders and diarrhea, but what you may not know is that it can also effectively lower your blood pressure.

In fact, Barberry leaf is regularly used to reduce edema in Iran and its bark is used to treat high blood pressure in France. Traditional Chinese medicine also commonly uses coptis and other plants containing berberine for treating heart ailments.

A combination of Chrysanthemum and Japanese Honeysuckle is also used to treat high blood pressure in traditional Chinese medicine.

Yarrow is also used for lowering blood pressure and relaxing blood vessels, although it is more commonly known to reduce fever and cure wounds.

Remember that you need to be very careful when taking a combination of herbs, over-the-counter medications, and prescription drugs.

You'll have to do some careful research before you try new herbs and be sure to take note of how your body reacts to it. You should also make sure the herbs don't interact negatively with any other medication you may be taking.

For example, there's plenty of argument going on about whether ginseng actually improves or worsens the condition of someone who has high blood pressure.

Perhaps the best thing for you to do before taking herbs and other medications is to consult your doctor and make sure it's safe.

What Part Does Potassium Play?

If you're concerned about your blood pressure, then you need to realize that your potassium intake and your blood pressure have an inverse relationship. This means that your blood pressure can rise as a result of low potassium intake.

Studies have shown that those who consume the recommended daily amount of potassium (4.7grams) have significantly lower blood pressure.

You take in potassium mainly from food sources like fresh fruits and vegetables, which is why it's very important for you to follow a healthy and well-balanced diet plan.

Many people are already aware that they need to minimize their sodium intake in order to control their blood pressure. But, it was only in 2005 when special focus was directed at the effects of potassium on our blood pressure. This was when more people finally became aware of how the sodium-potassium ratio in our body actually affects our blood pressure.

Dietary guidelines published in that year recommended an increase in the consumption of foods rich in potassium such as vegetables and fresh fruits.

A total of 32 trials were conducted to see just how effective potassium is in reducing blood pressure. In an analysis of those trials, supplementing with potassium was seen to reduce blood pressure by 4.4 mmHg and 2.25 mmHg (systolic/diastolic) in people who already have blood pressure.

Taking all of the test subjects into account, the average reduction in blood pressure was 3.1 mmHg and 2.0 mmHg.

A survey further confirmed the results of these trials when it showed that people who ate about 8.5 servings of fresh fruits and vegetables each day lowered their blood pressure by 7.2/2.8 mmHg.

What is it that makes potassium work so well against high blood pressure?

Well, potassium plays a major role in the synthesis of proteins in your body as well as the growth of your muscle tissues. It works inside all of your cells and helps maintain pH levels. It also acts as an electrolyte, which means it transmits electrical activity between your cells.

The activity of your heart and the contraction of your muscles depend largely on potassium. And because many of your body's activities are controlled by the activity of your muscles, potassium is therefore essential to maintain the normal functions of your body.

The problem is that a lot of people, especially in the Western countries, consume only about half of the recommended daily potassium intake.

You would do well to increase your intake of fresh fruits and vegetables to address this issue. Spinach, chard, and crimini mushrooms are excellent sources of potassium.

You may also get adequate amounts of potassium from fennel, mustard greens, kale, broccoli, Brussels sprouts, blackstrap molasses, bell peppers, eggplant, winter squash, tomatoes, summer squash, jackfruit, papaya, asparagus, turnip greens, shiitake mushrooms, celery, romaine lettuce, and prunes.

All types of meat are also excellent sources of potassium.

Of course, the best way to make sure you get adequate amounts of potassium each day is still to eat a healthy and well-balanced diet.

Taking in potassium in the recommended daily amount becomes even more important when you've been diagnosed with high blood pressure. Even if your blood pressure is still within normal levels, though, you'd do well to eat healthy.

The Food Factor

To make it easier for you to know what you should and shouldn't eat if you have high blood pressure, we have here a breakdown of what foods you should avoid and what you should consume more of.

What to Avoid

Generally speaking, people with high blood pressure need to avoid packaged foods, sugary foods, and red meat. You should also be careful about what you eat in restaurants when you have hypertension. Those whose blood pressure is still within normal levels are advised to take in no more than 2400mg of sodium each day. If you're already diagnosed with high blood pressure, however, the amount of sodium you can safely take in each day lowers to 1500mg.

If there are still packaged foods in your cupboard, take time to check the sodium content of each. You'll probably be shocked to see just how much the amount of sodium you consume from these packaged foods can add up. Remember that sodium is known to constrict your blood vessels, thus making it more difficult for blood to pass through smoothly. This is why sodium is a known contributor to hypertension and why you need to limit your sodium intake.

The good news is that it can be easy for you to prepare healthy meals for yourself and for your family. You may want to watch a few cooking shows so you'll get an idea on how to get started.

Eating at home is always preferable, of course, since restaurant food tend to have too much sodium in them. If you really need or want to eat out, then it may be a good idea to ask for a doggy bag at the outset so you can avoid consuming too much sodium in just one meal.

Where red meats are concerned, fats are the reason why you need to avoid them. Red meat usually puts fat into your veins and arteries, thus causing them to get clogged and making your blood pressure rise.

You don't really have to completely eliminate red meat and sugary foods from your diet. What's important is that you consume them in minimal amounts.

In fact, eating everything in moderation is generally a good idea, unless your doctor tells you otherwise.

What to Eat More Of

In order to keep your blood pressure at normal and healthy levels, you need to eat more fresh fruits and vegetables, low-fat dairy products, black beans, and fish. When you're craving for a hamburger, a black bean burger can be a delicious substitute.

And as you probably know by now, it's important to keep your stress level in check if you want to control your blood pressure. The good news is that there are certain foods that can help relax your arteries and lower your blood pressure.

A quick way to lower your blood pressure is by adding one or two teaspoons of apple cider vinegar to water. It may not really taste so good, but the results are surely worth the small sacrifice.

Take note, though, that if you're under medication for diabetes, you'll have to consult your doctor regarding apple cider vinegar intake.

Eating oatmeal for breakfast is also a good idea not only for losing weight, but also for delaying plaque build-up in your arteries.

If you crave something crunchy to eat, then celery is your best bet! It contains phytochemicals that relax your arterial walls and lower blood pressure.

Daily monitoring of your blood pressure is, of course, a must for making sure your numbers are always within a healthy range.

Living with High Blood Pressure

Once you're diagnosed with high blood pressure, you'll have to live with the condition for the rest of your life. That's because high blood pressure can't be cured, although it can be treated and managed.

A healthier lifestyle, medication, and continuing medical care will now be a normal part of your life.

When you treat the condition and your blood pressure normalizes as a result, that doesn't mean you can go back to your old habits. If you do, your blood pressure is bound to rise again and your condition may even worsen. What you need to do instead is strictly follow the treatment plan advised by your doctor and keep working to control your blood pressure for as long as you live.

Continuing medical care involves seeing your doctor for testing or routine check-ups as often as recommended after your initial testing and diagnosis.

Your doctor may make some adjustments to your treatment plan from time to time, based on the results of your regular check-ups. During each visit to your doctor, you shouldn't hesitate to ask any question about your treatment and lifestyle if you feel the need to.

Your doctor is likely to prescribe medication, depending on the severity of your condition. Be sure to take the prescribed medicines strictly according to your doctor's orders.

In case you have problems with regard to cost or side effects, don't just stop taking the medicines without informing your doctor. Rather, go see your doctor again and ask about alternative treatment options.

You may even want to discuss natural remedies for high blood pressure with him. There are several herbs and natural treatment methods that are known to help improve blood pressure. If your condition isn't that severe, these natural remedies may suffice.

You should also start adopting healthy habits once you're diagnosed with high blood pressure. This involves eating a well-balanced diet, exercising regularly, and maintaining your ideal weight.

If you are a smoker and a drinker, then you need to start limiting your alcohol intake and quit smoking. It would also be to your advantage if you learned how to manage stress better.

Develop a happy and optimistic outlook and learn some relaxation techniques such as yoga or meditation. For some people, something as simple as getting a massage or listening to music can effectively ease stress.

It would also be a good idea for you to learn how to measure your blood pressure on your own so you can keep track of the numbers at home.

You may ask your doctor to teach you how to measure your blood pressure. And every time you do, be sure to write down the measurements as well as the date and time you took the measurement.

Remember, you can't just treat high blood pressure and then ignore it.

It's something you'll have to manage for as long as you live, so it's best to do whatever you can to keep your blood pressure under control.

It can be a bit difficult to stick to the lifestyle changes you just made. But, you just have to think about the possible complications of high blood pressure and you'll surely appreciate your healthier lifestyle even more.

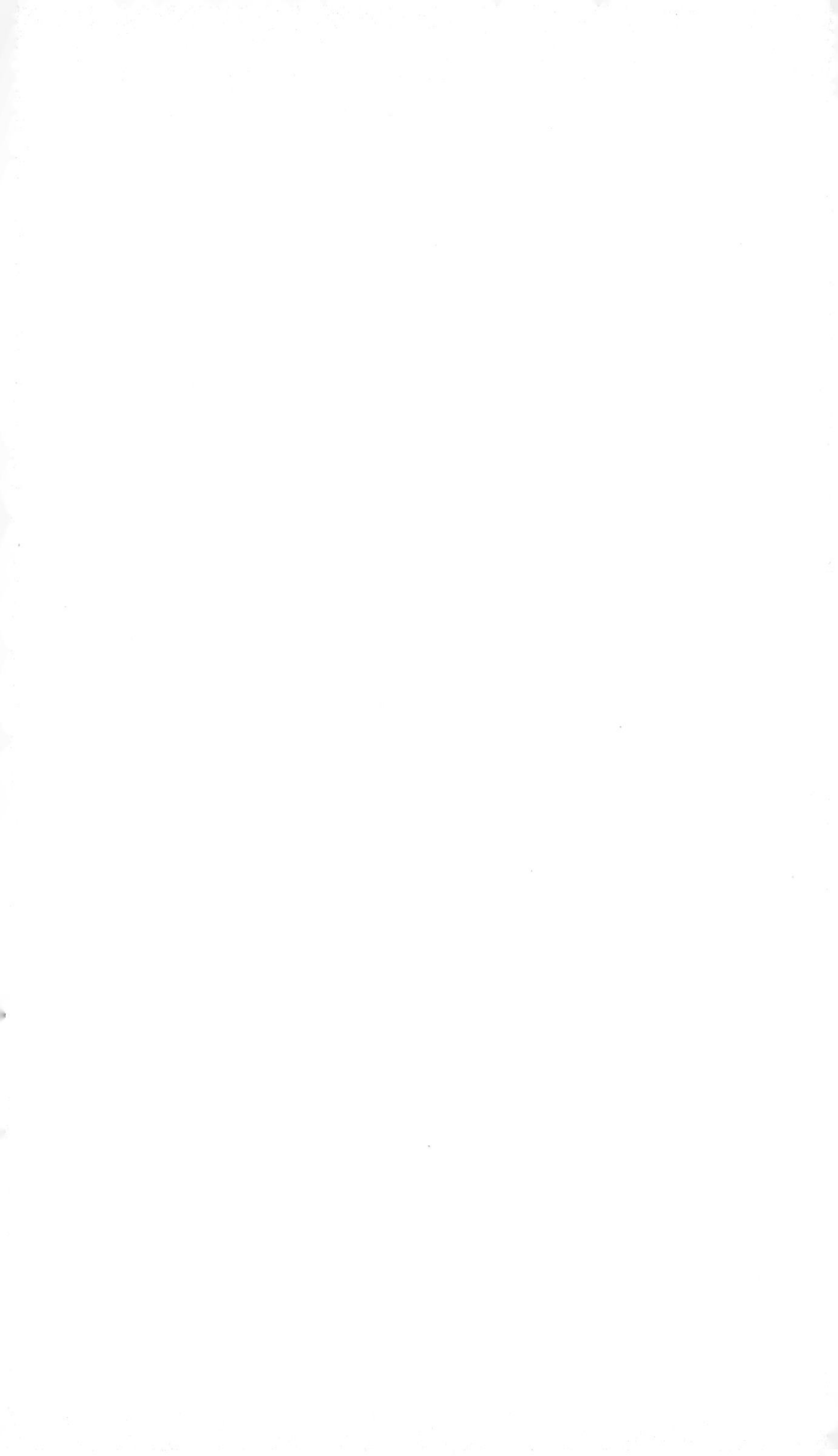

Printed in Great Britain
by Amazon